Miracle Epsom Salt:
Top 28 Epsom Salt Recipes

Table of content

Introduction

Epsom salt is something that everyone should have in his or her home. Recently it has become popular for its detox bath, but what people don't know is its ability to do so much more. There are literally hundreds of uses for Epsom salt through out the home and even outside the home in your garden.

Today we'll discuss the uses for Epsom Salt in regards to improving your health and enhancing your beauty. Epsom Salt has a strong history of being able to do these things and is proven to be safe and free from side effects unlike so many other products on the market today.

You can feel safe and comfortable investing both your time and your money in learning about and then putting together various Epsom Salt recipes for use in your home knowing that they will be not only effective, but also safe. The other great thing about Epsom Salt is how affordable it is. You won't spend hundreds of dollars on Epsom Salt and the other ingredients needed to put together these recipes. Instead you'll spend a fraction of the cost and get the same or even better results than other similar products.

Chapter 1 – What is Epsom Salt and Why Does it Work?

Epsom Salt gets its name from the salt like or bitter taste that is similar to salt, but it actually isn't salt at all. Instead, it is the compound of the minerals magnesium and sulfate. It was first found in England in the small town of Surrey. It was found in a spring there that was a saline spring called Epsom Spring, hence now we have the name, Epsom salt.

The magnesium found in Epsom salt is very beneficial to the human body. It can help with a number of different things like the reduction of inflammation and prevention of artery clogging. It can also help to improve overall muscle function as well as nerve communication. Studies have also shown that magnesium helps control and regulate enzymes in the body. Magnesium is extremely effective when absorbed through the skin, but can also be effective other ways.

Epsom salt also contains sulfates, which are also extremely helpful to the body. Sulfates generally help the body absorb and breakdown other minerals and nutrients that the body receives either through food, vitamins, the sun, etc. It can also help with getting rid of any toxins in the body through the colon, liver, etc. Finally, studies are showing us that sulfates can help to give relief to those that experience intense or even migraine headaches.

It is important that you look at the quality and grade of the Epsom salt you purchase. There are several different brands out there that would sell you a cheaper product that is low quality. You will get what you pay for. You will want to make sure you buy high quality Epsom salt in order to see the results you want when it comes to your health and beauty. Even if you are going to use it around your home or garden, you'll want high quality Epsom salt as well.

Look for things like pharmaceutical-grade in order to ensure that you are getting a high quality product. You can also look at reviews from other customers to see what they say and how they have used to product. If they have used the product for the same type of things you plan to and saw good results, you can rest assured that it will work well for you, too.

Chapter 2 – DIY Epsom Salt Recipes for Improved Health

Your health and the health of those you love should be the number one priority for you, and if using Epsom salt in your life can help improve that, it should be in your home. Here are some great easy and convenient ways to use Epsom salt to improve your health.

You'll notice that some of these recipes and uses can be combined or will be combined as you do them. For example, if you take an Epsom Salt Bath, you'll also relieve any muscle aches you have simply by allowing the Epsom salt to absorb into your skin through the water. If you aren't experiencing any muscle aches, at the time you take a bath, you won't get this added benefit, but I don't know about anyone else, I always seem to have at least a muscle ache or two somewhere in my body that could use a little help.

Epsom Salt Bath

This is honestly like going to the spa; only you're going to do it in your own home after a long day at work or a long day taking care of the kids. It's extremely relaxing and will be a great way for you to allow the magnesium and sulfates in Epsom salt to absorb naturally in to your skin. Here's how you do it:

Simply start running the warm bath water. It doesn't matter how hot you run the water, so do it at a temperature that is comfortable to you. As the water runs, add a cup of Epsom salt to the bath water so that it dissolves into the water as the bathtub is filling.

Once the tub is full and the salt has dissolved, get in and enjoy yourself. You can stay in an Epsom salt bath as long as you like.

Ache and Pain Relief Bath

The Epsom salt bath is extremely nice after you've experienced a long day and feel like you need the spa treatment, but if you've ever spent a long day at the gym, or if your work requires heavy lifting, then you know what's it like to be extremely sore and tired in a different way.

An Epsom salt bath can be extremely helpful in giving relief for this kind of ailment, too. If you are experiencing muscle aches and pains, then put yourself in an Epsom salt bath to experience the relief you need.

The bath is essentially the same. Start the water, dissolve a cup of Epsom salt into it and wait for it to dissolve. Once the salt has dissolved and the tub is full, enjoy the bath to help take away your pain. This is a great way for you to enjoy the bath, while also speeding up your recovery process.

Epsom Salt Foot Bath

If you don't feel like taking an entire bath after work, consider just a footbath. There are plenty of people that are on their feet all day at work or even at home doing things around the house. This makes for a difficult and tiring job by the end of the day. You don't need any intense equipment, just a deep container that you can soak your feet in while you sit on the couch.

Get a container a fill it full of nice warm water. The water doesn't need to be hot, just comfortable for you to soak your feet. Dissolve a few tablespoons of Epsom salt in the water. The more water you have, you may want to throw in an extra tablespoon of Epsom salt. Start with two or three and see how you feel. If you are getting the desired effect, you are okay. If you aren't satisfied, it's probably because you need a little more Epsom salt. Let the salt dissolve in the water.

Soak your feet for thirty minutes to an hour. You'll start to feel relief immediately!

Fight Constipation

If you are experiencing constipation and you need some relief, you can turn to Epsom salt to help. Of course there are plenty of over the counter remedies that can help, too, but when there is a natural alternative that won't give you any other side effects, it's nice to know Epsom salt can help. You can simply mix a teaspoon of Epsom salt with eight to ten ounces of water. Let it dissolve into the water before drinking to ensure that you get all the salt. Then drink up. You should start to feel relief within an hour.

The magnesium combined with the sulfates will loosen things up and help give you some relief.

Epsom Salt Detox

This is a little bit similar to the last use of Epsom salt, but with more benefits. There are so many over the counter drugs that you can buy that are advertised as colon cleanses. The problem with these is that they are filled with artificial ingredients and fillers. The whole point of a colon cleanse is to get rid of things just like that, so why would you put them in into you body just to get rid of them. It seems like this weird oxymoron. Instead you can use the same drink mix of one teaspoon and eight ounces of water to flush out your colon when needed.

It is important that you discuss a colon cleanse with your doctor before performing it and when considering to perform on a regular basis. Some people who take other medications can react adversely to a colon cleanse, so make sure you are a good candidate for a colon cleanse before performing one or performing them regularly.

Using Epsom Salt to Help with Hangovers

We all have the tendency to let loose every once in a while and when that happens we sure regret it the next day. There are tons of remedies for hangovers out there and some are better than others. Epsom salt to help you get back on your feet is one of the better ones out there.

Hangovers are the result of two things – dehydration and toxins in the body. Dehydration can be easily solved by drinking water. Step one that's basically free and easy for you to accomplish on your own. Step two is a little trickier – getting rid of the toxins. Luckily, that's where Epsom salts can step in and do the work for you.

Epsom salt has sulfates, which we've learned can help to break down those toxins quickly and efficiently, which will get them out of your system; thus helping you to feel better and back to feeling normal.

The best way to accomplish this is drinking a glass of Epsom salt water like we've been discussing. It's quick and efficient for getting the Epsom salt into your system and working in your favor. You can also take an Epsom salt bath, which we discussed earlier, which will absorb the salt into your skin; it just will take longer to go into effect.

It is important to remember that salts, even Epsom salt, and does work against your hydration, so keep that water going all day long in order to combat the dehydration from the night before.

Help a Bruise Heal Faster

When you get a nasty looking bruise, the last thing you want it to do is linger. This is especially true if it is in a location that is easily visible to others. You want it to heal and be less noticeable as quickly as possible. There are expensive creams and make-up that people often try to hide bruises, but those rarely work, and make-up often rubs off after just a short time.

Instead, you want something that is actually working under the skin to help the damaged tissue start to heal sooner, thus making your skin appear normal. Thus you aren't hiding the bruise, you're working to make it better. See the difference?

This is accomplished with the help of Epsom salt and cold water. You'll want to make a cold compress with the cold water and two tablespoons of Epsom salt. Then take the cold compress and gently place it on the bruised skin. Hold it there for at least ten minutes, but up to thirty. Once you notice that the compress is no longer cold, it will have lost its effectiveness.

You can repeat the process with a new compress, using cold water again, but wait at least thirty minutes in between applications. You can also do it once in the morning and again at night.

Use Epsom Salt to Help You Fall Asleep

Epsom salt is a great way to help you unwind at night. If you find that you are the kind of person that tends to lie awake at night for hours or even an hour before eventually falling asleep, consider using Epsom salt to help you relax and unwind before bed.

Studies have shown that people who use an Epsom salt bath before bed are relaxed and in a state that is ready for bed when the clock says it's bedtime. Rather than tossing and turning for thirty minutes or an hour, those who spend twenty or thirty minutes in a Epsom salt bath report that they have no trouble falling asleep.

Additionally remember all the other benefits of an Epsom salt bath. It's like knocking out two birds with one stone (or ten birds with one stone).

Combat Stress with Epsom Salt

Stress is a huge concern for a lot of people. There is a point of healthy stress in our lives that is okay to have and important to keep us motivated each day; however, there is also a point at which we have to say we are overstressed and it is unhealthy. It is at that point that we have to say we need to do something different.

Lots of people spend hundreds of dollars on stress health coaching, spa days, etc. in order to help combat their stress levels. Although these things may be helpful, a nice Epsom salt bath may be all you need on a regular basis to reduce your stress level enough to keep it healthy. It sure doesn't hurt to try it and see what it does to your overall mood and levels of energy.

For so many people just a nice warm bath without any interruptions is a wonderful thought. Now add on top of that, the added benefits of Epsom salt. It's simple, easy and costs almost nothing to throw a cup of salt into the bath while you're in there; however the added benefits are through the roof. You'll feel stronger and your load will feel lighter when you're done.

Epsom Salt Sunburn Treatment

We all get sunburned on occasion and so do our family members. There are many products out there to help with sunburns, but like so many other things we've talked about, how many of them are filled with things we can't pronounce and don't know what we're putting on our bodies. When we put things on our bodies those products are absorbed into our skin and bloodstream. Are we okay with that?

Instead, it's so nice to know we have the option of using something with only two ingredients, one of which is Epsom salt. Epsom salt is effective on sunburns because it actually has an anti-inflammatory effect on the skin and pulls the heat out of the burn.

To make a treatment to the following:

Grab a spray bottle and mix together a cup of water, you can start with warm water if it's easier and add two tablespoons of Epsom salt. Let the salt dissolve into the water (hence the warm water). Once the salt is dissolved it is ready for use.

You can keep it in the fridge to keep it cold if you prefer, but it doesn't need to be. Spray on any sunburned skin to help. It can be applied as often as necessary.

Improve Your Heart Health

For those with a risk of heart disease either because they've been told that by a doctor, or because they have a history in their family, Epsom salt is a great way to help improve and prevent future heart problems. Of course it isn't the only way to improve heart health – diet and exercise are important, too – but using Epsom salt in addition to these other factors can help to improve heart health that much more.

Because Epsom salt will help to increase your blood circulation and prevent arteries from clogging, you know you're on the right path to improved health. It also helps to stop blood clots, which will lower the risk of heart attacks as well.

Adding an Epsom salt bath once a week into your life can help with these benefits by letting your body absorb the magnesium and sulfates.

Epsom Salt for Diabetics and Potential Diabetics

Studies are showing that Epsom salt can and does help with insulin regulation as well. This also has to do with the magnesium and sulfate properties in Epsom salt and how they react with the insulin in the body. When the two combine they work together in such a way that helps the insulin be more effective and work properly.

For people with diabetes, this could be a huge breakthrough. It may not be a cure for them, but it could help with regulation or with their severity. Drinking a glass of Epsom salt water is much cheaper than most of the insulin shots they have to purchase both with and without insurance.

This can also help with potential diabetics. If you run the risk of getting diabetes, this is a way you can help yourself bring that risk level back down. Start drinking a glass of Epsom water (1 teaspoon to eight ounces of water), every day to help your insulin levels regulate themselves.

Epsom Salt to Help with Gout

Epsom salt will not cure gout, but it will help with the pain or the discomfort of gout. It can help because the Epsom salt will help to bring down the inflammation caused by gout, thus reducing the pain and uncomfortable nature.

Find a basin or container large enough that you'll be able to soak your affected joint and fill it full of warm/hot water. Add upwards of a tablespoon (depending on the size of the container) to the water. You want the water to be comfortable, but the hotter the better, so it will stay warm for as long as possible. Ideally you want to soak your joint for thirty minutes and have the water still be warm.

Epsom Salt to Get Rid of Foot Odor

We've talked about soaking your feet before in an Epsom salt footbath before, but that was for aching feet. This is just another great use and benefit of Epsom salt. If you create a footbath for your feet, you can also remove foot odor. Depending on how strong the foot odor is, you may want to use more Epsom salt.

It is recommended that you pour half a cup of Epsom salt for a foot odor bath. Then soak your feet for at least ten minutes to help with any foot odor problems. Of course you can always soak them for longer!

Epsom Salt to Help with Splinter Removal

At this point, you might be a little skeptical, but it really works. Wherever you have a splinter, you can soak it in a small Epsom salt bath and it will help to bring out the splinter. It may not draw it out completely depending on how embedded the splinter is, but it will start the process for you.

Can you imagine how great this is for parents of little ones? Instead of having to dig around with tweezers for a splinter, you can soak the affected area for a few minutes and then make the process virtually painless for a small child.

Epsom Salt for Sprains

I know this is starting to sound redundant, so we'll keep it short, but get yourself ready to take an Epsom salt bath unless you can just soak the sprain in a smaller bath by itself.

For a sprain, you may want to add upwards of two cups to the bath water to help with the swelling, too. It will depend on how bad the sprain is – you can be the judge of how much Epsom salt you want to add.

Epsom Salt for Athlete's Foot

Again, you can soak your foot or feet in a full Epsom salt bath (because at this point, why wouldn't you just take a full body bath), and enjoy the benefits of helping with your symptoms. It won't cure your athlete's foot, but it will help to give you some relief.

Epsom Salt for Toenail Fungus

Okay this one isn't just for the symptoms of your feet, but it will treat it, too. So create a footbath with 3-5 T of Epsom salt and soak your toes. In order to fully treat and cure them, you'll want to try and do this three times through out the day.

Epsom Salt and an Ice Bath

Lots of athletes use ice baths after workouts or injuries to help with inflammation. The best thing about Epsom salt is that like ice, it can combat inflammation as well. So putting the two together, you can really fight inflammation if you're experiencing an injury and help speed recovery times.

If you are going to start an ice bath, proceed with your ice bath as normal, simply add four cups of Epsom salt sprinkled through out. Ease your way into the ice bath, good luck!

Chapter 3 – DIY Epsom Salt Recipes for Improved and Enhanced Beauty

Sometimes it's nice to have some alternative ways to enhance your beauty rather than spending hundreds of dollars on beauty products. We all have our favorite beauty products, and they may cost a fair amount of money. We also like to pamper ourselves every once in a while. But what if there were products that we could make with Epsom salt that were just as good as our expensive ones or ways to pamper ourselves at home with Epsom salt that were far less expensive and gave us just as good of results? Wouldn't you jump at the opportunity? Here are some great alternatives and great options to consider when it comes to beauty.

Epsom Salt Food Scrub

I know I hate it when the soles of my feet dry up and get cracked. It's those times of the year that I feel like getting a pedicure just to have the products they use soften up my feet and help get rid of all the dry skin. If you aren't one to spend the money on pedicures, you still might by food scrubs or food lotions, too, and they can be just as pricey. So here's a great alternative recipe using Epsom salt that you can make at home and have for a really long time!

Ingredients

2 C Epsom salt

½ C almond oil

2 t liquid castile soap

25-30 drops of your favorite essential oil

Directions

Use a medium sized mixing bowl and combine all the ingredients together, adding any essential oils you plan to use last. When you add the essential oils, it's recommended that you add them a little at a time until you get the scent you want. Some can be a little stronger than others, so remember that you can always add more, but can't take the oils back out once you've added them in.

To use the scrub, just apply it to your feet with a small brush or cloth. Let it sit for a minute or two to exfoliate your pores and pull off the dry skin. Then rinse off the scrub using warm water.

The best way to store your Epsom Salt Foot Scrub is in a jar that has an airtight lid. This will help it last upwards of a year. You'll start to feel its effectiveness go after six months though, so it is best if used within six months. If you don't think you'll use the full recipe within six months, it's best to half the recipe or make it and give half to a friend for a gift!

*Note you can also make a combination of several essential oils to make a floral scent or combination of scents that you like. It's completely up to you how you want to scent your scrub.

Epsom Salt Eye Wash

The eyes are such a tricky part of the body. We want them to be stunning and noticeable all the time, but as we grow older they constantly seem to have problems. Epsom salt is a great tool to help with eye health, both as we grow older and to encourage good eye health overall.

Just a few things that Epsom salt can help with include cataracts and conjunctivitis as well as styes. It's important that you use the eyewash regularly to help with overall eye health as well.

Take a small glass of warm water and dissolve a teaspoon of Epsom salt. Watch carefully to make sure all the salt is dissolved. Once it's dissolved you can apply it directly around the eyes as an eyewash with a cotton swab, cotton ball, pad, etc. You can also soak a washcloth with the salt water and use it like a warm compress over your eyes.

Epsom Salt Hair Volumizer

Sometimes you might notice that your hair feels different after you shower or blow-dry your hair. It might feel like it's heavy or even feels like it's extremely oily even though you just washed it that morning. This is a normal occurrence for many women and it actually comes back to the fact that they are using store bought shampoo and conditioner filled with additives and fillers that use oils and other things we don't even understand.

Although you can change this by making your own shampoo and conditioner, that's a book for another day and time. To solve this problem with a simple fix and solution, you can use a quick Epsom salt Volumizer that will help to give you some volume, which combats the heavy feeling you have, while also cleaning out any toxins and oils or grease that your shampoo or conditioner may have left behind.

Here's the recipe:

½ C Organic Conditioner

½ C Epsom salt

Instructions

In a small bowl mix together the conditioner and the Epsom salt. Once it is well combined you can apply it directly onto your hair or you can store it in an airtight container for later use.

When you are ready to use, put the conditioner into your hair just like you normally would, you can and probably want to do this prior to getting in the shower. Then leave the conditioner in your hair for twenty-thirty minutes. After twenty or thirty minutes, rinse the conditioner out of your hair with warm water. For optimal results, you can repeat this on a weekly basis.

*Note: You can make more or less of this product based on how much you need for your length of hair. Just note that the parts of conditioner to Epsom salt are equal. You can also make it and store it for up to a month at a time if you plan to do it weekly.

Epsom Salt for Chapped Lips

Dry or chapped lips are extremely annoying and not to mention painful when they crack and bleed. Oh and it's also pretty embarrassing, too. You aren't going to impress anyone with dry, chapped or cracked and bleeding lips. We all want lips that look healthy and lush.

It's a pain to buy chapstick on a constant basis, especially when you constantly lose it or have to keep track of five different sticks in different locations so you have one on hand wherever you might need one. Instead, turn to Epsom salt for the answer. Epsom salt can give you healthy lips, because it will get rid of the dead skin and help to keep your lips full and beautiful.

Here's how you do it:

Ingredients

2 t Epsom salt

2 T Coconut Oil

2 T Cacao Butter

Instructions

Mix together all the ingredients in a small or medium mixing bowl. Make sure everything is well combined. It is ready then for immediate use or you can store it in an airtight container for up to a month.

When ready to use, apply a small layer on both your top and bottom lip. Gently rub it into your lips using both your fingers and rubbing your lips together. You'll want as much of the lip balm to actually rub into your lips. You may have a little excess, which you can wipe away after a few minutes of rubbing. Over time, you'll get a feel for how much to apply in the first place and hopefully you won't have any excess.

Epsom Salt Facial

A day at the spa to get a facial is just one of those things that sounds so relaxing sometimes. However, for some of us, that just isn't budget friendly. We love the idea, but our wallet, shakes its head in disgust. So when you have the idea of getting a facial, give this great little recipe a try.

It's simple and affordable, while also giving you that fresh feeling of just spending a day at the spa. The only part about it that's hard is that you have to do the work yourself and aren't pampered on by someone else. But you do get some great results for your face, so it's still a win there!

Here's what you need and how to do it:

Ingredients

½ - 1 t Epsom salt

Your choice of Organic Face Cleansing Cream

Instructions

Get a medium sized bowl and mix together a normal amount of your favorite face cleansing cream. When we say normal, this is the amount that it would take to cover your face and neck. Then add in the Epsom salt and mix the two together until they are well combined. You can choose just how much Epsom salt to add. For people with sensitive skin, it's recommended to add less.

Once the mixture is mixed well, it is ready for use. Apply it gently to the skin and rub across your face and neck. The salt will help to exfoliate and clean out your pores more than the regular cleansing cream. You can leave on the facial as long as your regular cream instructed, but don't leave it on any longer.

Rinse your face with cold water when you are finished. You should see and feel immediate results after rinsing.

Epsom Salt Skin Exfoliator

We talked a little about a facial exfoliator, but sometimes you need it more than just on your face. You can use this recipe anywhere, but also on your face.

While you are in the shower or the bathtub, use a small handful of Epsom salt with about a tablespoon of olive oil. You can rub this mixture all over any dead skin or just over your wet skin. This will exfoliate your skin while also softening. After it sits for a minute, rinse with warm water.

Epsom Salt to Get Rid of Blackheads

Blackheads are extremely annoying and any products you buy from the store are full of chemicals. So instead, consider creating something with Epsom salt that will help with your skin, while also getting rid of blackheads.

Ingredients

2 t Epsom salt

6 drops iodine

1 C boiling water

Instructions

Mix everything together in the boiling water until the Epsom salt dissolves. Let it cool before applying to your face or neck. Once the mixture is cool you can apply it with a cotton ball, tissue, cotton swab, etc.

Epsom Salt to Breakdown Hairspray

For those of us who use hairspray on a regular basis, it really never feels like we can get it completely out. We may wash our hair, but there always feels like a residue of hairspray is still there.

Epsom salt is a great way to ensure that the hairspray is finally gone and our hair is completely clean.

Ingredients

½ gallon of water

½ C lemon juice

½ C Epsom salt

Instructions

Combine everything in a bucket or container with a lid and let it sit for 24 hours. After 24 hours, it is ready for use. Using a ladle or a cup, pour the mixture through your hair while it is still dry. Leave it in your hair for twenty-thirty minutes before showering.   After twenty-thirty minutes, shower and use shampoo to remove.

Epsom Salt for Intense Exfoliation

Sometimes you just want something a little stronger. This is a recipe for just that. It isn't the exfoliation you do a daily or even a few times a week. This is for when you really want to see a difference. This shouldn't be done on any broken skin or if you any irritated skin either.

Ingredients

1 C Epsom Salt

¼ C Coconut Oil

2 drops Lavender Essential Oil (or another favorite essential oil)

Instructions

Mix together all three ingredients in a small mixing bowl until they are well combined. It is ready for immediate use or you can store it in an airtight container until you are ready to use.

When you are ready to use it, rub it over the skin gently. It should rub into the skin like a lotion.

Conclusion

Epsom salt is a great way to introduce a natural healing and enhancing benefit into your home. It is cheap and affordable while also giving you wonderful benefits you would have never thought imaginable.

The uses are truly amazing and we didn't even begin to cover all of them in this book. There are so many more that the possibilities are endless. You'll love the fact that you have a new power and ability to bring a natural occurring mineral into your home that is safe to use while also having so many uses and benefits.

You won't ever regret the day you started using Epsom salt.

FREE Bonus Reminder

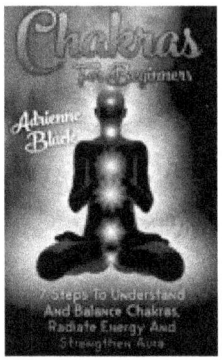

If you have not grabbed it yet, please go ahead and download your special bonus E book *"Chakras for Beginners. 7 Steps To Understand And Balance Chakras, Radiate Energy, And Strengthen Aura"*.

Simply Click the Button Below

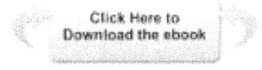

OR Go to This Page

http://lifehacksworld.com/free

BONUS #2: More Free & Discounted Books & Products

Do you want to receive more Free/Discounted Books or Products?

We have a mailing list where we send out our new Books or Products when they go free or with a discount on Amazon. Click on the link below to sign up for Free & Discount Book & Product Promotions.

=> **Sign Up for Free & Discount Book & Product Promotions** <=

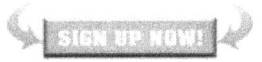

OR Go to this URL

http://zbit.ly/1WBb1Ek